DEFEAT WEIGHT

DEFEAT WEIGHT

The Back Entryway to Weight Misfortune

By

KEMP NOBLE

DISCLAIMER

Copyright © by Kemp Noble 2023. All rights reserved

Before this this document is duplicated or reproduced in any manner, the publisher's consent must be gained.

DEFEAT WEIGHT

Therefore, the consent within can neither be stored electronically, transferred nor kept in a database. Neither in part or in full can the document can be copied, scanned, faxed, or retained without approval from the publisher or creator.

TABLE OF CONTENT

•I defeated weight: Achieving Sustainable Weight Loss through Comprehensive Nutrition/exercises

Chapter 5

•I maintained my weight: Patience And Consistency

DEFEAT WEIGHT
INTRODUCTION

Welcome to an exploration that transcends the conventional narratives surrounding weight loss, inviting you to consider an alternative perspective — the back doorway to achieving lasting and transformative results in your health journey.

In the vast landscape of wellness, weight loss is a prevalent and often challenging goal for many individuals. Traditional approaches, such as dieting and intense exercise regimens, dominate the discourse, but our exploration seeks to broaden the horizon. Beyond the well-trodden paths lies a less-explored route, the back doorway, which holds the promise of unconventional yet effective strategies.

In this journey, we will navigate through the intricacies of weight loss, acknowledging that it is not merely a physical endeavor but a holistic transformation encompassing mind, body, and lifestyle. The back doorway represents a metaphorical entry point to this comprehensive understanding, urging us to look beyond quick fixes and embrace sustainable, long-term solutions.

Holistic health practices, encompassing nutrition, physical activity, mental well-being, and lifestyle choices, form the foundation of our exploration. We will delve into the interconnected nature of these elements, recognizing that true weight loss success stems from a harmonious balance rather than isolated efforts. This broader perspective encourages us to view weight loss not as a singular goal but as an integral part of a lifelong journey toward overall well-being.

Unearthing the secrets behind defeating weight requires a shift in mindset — from viewing weight loss as a destination to approaching it as a continuous process of self-discovery and improvement. Through the back doorway, we open ourselves to innovation and adaptability, acknowledging that there is no one-size-fits-all solution. Each

DEFEAT WEIGHT

individual's path to weight loss is unique, and our exploration will provide the tools to tailor strategies to personal needs and preferences.

As we traverse this uncharted territory, we will encounter diverse modalities, from mindful eating practices to

personalized fitness routines and stress management techniques. The back doorway beckons us to explore the benefits of holistic health, emphasizing not only the physical aspects of weight loss but also the mental and emotional dimensions that contribute to sustainable change.

Ultimately, our journey through the back doorway seeks to empower you with knowledge, inspire a shift in perspective, and equip you with practical tools to defeat weight on your terms. Join us as we embark on a transformative exploration, opening doors to a healthier, more balanced life that extends beyond the confines of conventional weight loss approaches. The back doorway awaits, inviting you to

DEFEAT WEIGHT

step into a realm of holistic well-being and lasting change.

Chapter 1

My old friend (food): Your body Needs Food

Food plays a multifaceted and indispensable role in the human body, influencing various physiological processes and contributing to overall health and well-being. The importance of food stems from its ability to supply essential nutrients, serve as an energy source, support cellular function, and impact key aspects of bodily health.

Nutrient Supply

Food serves as the primary source of essential nutrients, including carbohydrates, proteins, fats, vitamins, and minerals. These nutrients are the building blocks necessary for the proper functioning of the body. For instance, proteins are crucial for tissue repair and growth, while vitamins and minerals play vital roles in enzyme function, immune system support, and maintaining a balance of bodily functions.

Energy Source

Carbohydrates, fats, and proteins, collectively known as macronutrients, are the body's fuel sources. Through complex metabolic processes, the body converts these nutrients into energy, providing the necessary fuel for daily activities, from basic bodily functions to physical exercise.

Cellular Function

Nutrients obtained from food are utilized by cells for various functions, such as building and repairing tissues, synthesizing enzymes and hormones, and maintaining the integrity of cell membranes. This cellular activity is essential for growth, development, and the ongoing maintenance of bodily structures.

Metabolism

Food intake significantly influences metabolic processes, including the metabolism of nutrients and the regulation of energy balance. A well-balanced diet supports healthy metabolism, contributing to weight management and the prevention of metabolic disorders.

Immune System Support

Certain nutrients, such as vitamins (e.g., vitamin C, vitamin D) and minerals (e.g., zinc), play a crucial role in supporting the immune system. Adequate nutrition enhances the body's ability to defend against infections and illnesses, promoting overall health.

Brain Function

The mind is a fairly metabolically lively organ that calls for a consistent delivery of vitamins to characteristic optimally.

Nutrients like omega-3 fatty acids, antioxidants, and certain vitamins are associated with cognitive function, memory, and mental well-being.

Bone Health

Calcium and vitamin D, obtained from food sources, are essential for maintaining strong and healthy bones. Proper nutrition during childhood and adulthood contributes to bone development and helps prevent conditions like osteoporosis.

Digestive Health

Dietary fiber, found abundantly in fruits, vegetables, and whole grains, is crucial for maintaining a healthy digestive system. It aids in digestion, prevents constipation, and helps the boom of useful intestine bacteria.

Blood Sugar Regulation

Balanced and nutritious meals contribute to the regulation of blood sugar levels. This is particularly important for individuals with conditions like diabetes, where maintaining stable blood sugar is critical for overall health.

Hydration

While not classified as a traditional "food," water is a vital component of a healthy diet. Proper hydration supports digestion, nutrient absorption,

DEFEAT WEIGHT

temperature regulation, and overall bodily function.

In summary, the importance of food extends far beyond mere sustenance. A well-balanced and varied diet is

paramount for maintaining optimal health, preventing nutritional deficiencies, and promoting longevity. Understanding the multifaceted role of food empowers individuals to make informed choices that

DEFEAT WEIGHT

positively impact their overall well-being.

Chapter 2

Why my body longs for food: Over-crave and over-starvation

Overeating habits can be influenced by various factors, including emotional triggers (stress, boredom), environmental cues (food availability, portion sizes), social influences, hormonal imbalances, and a lack of mindful eating practices. Understanding and addressing these factors can help in managing and preventing overeating.

Let's delve deeper into these factors

Emotional Triggers

Emotional states, which include stress, boredom, or sadness, can cause overeating as people search for consolation or distraction via food.

Environmental Cues

DEFEAT WEIGHT

The physical environment plays a crucial role. Abundant food availability, larger portion sizes, and easy access to high-calorie snacks can contribute to overeating.

Social Influences

Social situations, peer pressure, or cultural norms can influence eating habits. For example, social events centered around food may encourage overconsumption.

Hormonal Imbalances

DEFEAT WEIGHT

Hormones like ghrelin and leptin, which regulate hunger and satiety, can be influenced by factors like inadequate sleep, leading to disrupted appetite control.

Inattentiveness

Lack of awareness during meals, such as eating quickly or multitasking, can result in overeating.

Chapter 3

How I put on weight: Excessive Calories/medical conditions

Excessive food intake can lead to weight gain primarily due to an imbalance between the calories consumed and the calories expended by the body. When you regularly consume more calories than your body needs for daily activities and basic functions, the excess energy is stored as fat. Here is why….

Caloric Surplus

Consuming more calories than your body requires creates a surplus. These extra calories are stored as fat, leading to an increase in body weight.

Energy Storage

The body stores excess calories primarily in the form of adipose tissue (fat). This stored energy serves as a reserve for times when caloric intake is insufficient.

Metabolism and Activity Levels

If your metabolic rate (the rate at which your body burns calories at rest) remains relatively constant and your physical activity levels do not compensate for the excess calorie intake, weight gain occurs.

Genetic Factors

Individual genetic factors also play a role in how the body stores and utilizes energy. Some people may be genetically predisposed to store excess calories as fat more efficiently.

Hormonal Influences

Hormones, such as insulin, play a role in regulating metabolism and fat storage. Diets high in refined sugars and processed foods can lead to insulin spikes, promoting fat storage.

Health Conditions

Certain medical conditions or medications may affect

DEFEAT WEIGHT

metabolism and contribute to
weight gain.

Chapter 4

I defeated weight: Achieving Sustainable Weight Loss through Comprehensive Nutrition/exercises

Embarking on a journey to lose weight involves adopting a comprehensive approach that encompasses various aspects of nutrition, lifestyle, and mindset. This guide aims to provide a broad understanding of key principles for sustainable weight loss through nutritional adjustments and proper exercises.

Understanding Caloric Balance

Begin by grasping the concept of caloric balance - consuming fewer calories than your body expends. This forms the foundation of weight loss. Calculate your daily caloric needs based on factors like age, gender, activity level, and health status.

Nutrient-Rich Foods

Prioritize nutrient-dense foods to ensure your body receives essential vitamins and minerals. Include a colorful array of fruits, vegetables, lean proteins, whole grains, and low-fat dairy in your diet. These foods not only provide necessary nutrients but also contribute to a feeling of fullness.

Meal Planning and Portion Control

Effective weight management involves planning balanced meals.

DEFEAT WEIGHT

This helps in avoiding impulsive, unhealthy choices. Additionally, practice portion control to prevent overeating. Be mindful of serving sizes to align with your caloric goals.

Hydration

Hydrate your body with water, herbal teas, and other low-calorie beverages. Adequate hydration not only supports overall health but can also help control hunger and prevent unnecessary snacking.

Minimizing Processed Foods

Limit the intake of processed and refined foods, which often contain added sugars, unhealthy fats, and excess

sodium. Opt for whole, unprocessed alternatives to fuel your body with quality nutrients.

Establishing Regular Eating Patterns

Set consistent meal times to regulate your metabolism. Avoid skipping meals, as this can lead to increased hunger and potentially unhealthy food choices. Regular eating patterns contribute to stable energy levels throughout the day.

Balancing Healthy Fats and Proteins

Incorporate assets of wholesome fats, consisting of avocados, nuts, seeds, and olive oil, in moderation. Balance your diet with lean protein sources to support muscle health and promote a sense of satiety.

DEFEAT WEIGHT

Reducing Added Sugars

Cut back on added sugars found in sweets, sugary beverages, and processed snacks. Opt for herbal assets of sweetness, inclusive of fruits, to fulfill your candy tooth.

Mindful Eating

Cultivate a conscious method of consuming with the aid of taking note of starvation and fullness cues. This practice fosters a healthier relationship with food and helps prevent overindulgence.

Quality Sleep and Stress Management

Prioritize sufficient and quality sleep, as inadequate sleep can impact weight management. Additionally, practice stress-reducing techniques, as stress can influence eating habits and contribute to weight gain.

Physical Activity (core)

Adopting a holistic lifestyle that combines a diverse and nutritious diet with regular, varied physical activities, including a blend of aerobic exercises and strength

DEFEAT WEIGHT

training, serves as a multifaceted
foundation for

promoting overall health and
pursuing sustainable weight
management goals. This
integrative approach supports not
only physical well-being but also
contributes to a comprehensive
sense of vitality and fitness.

Chapter 5

I maintained my weight: Patience And Consistency

· Maintaining weight through patience and consistency involves adopting habits that promote a healthy and balanced lifestyle.

Establish Sustainable Habits:

•Cultivate long-term habits rather than relying on short-term solutions.

DEFEAT WEIGHT

Focus on making gradual, sustainable modifications to your food regimen and lifestyle.
•Celebrate small victories and stay committed to your health journey

Support System:
•Surround yourself with a supportive network of friends or family who encourage your healthy habits.
Share your goals and progress to reinforce your commitment,

DEFEAT WEIGHT

Patient:

- Understand that maintaining weight is an ongoing process. Weight fluctuations are normal, and patience is key to sustaining long-term success.

Consultation with Professionals

- For personalized advice tailored to your unique health needs and circumstances, always consult with a healthcare professional or a registered dietitian. They can provide guidance and support on your weight loss journey.

DEFEAT WEIGHT

•Remember, achieving and maintaining a healthy weight involves embracing a holistic lifestyle that nourishes your body, mind, and spirit.

www.ingramcontent.com/pod-product-compliance
Lightning Source LLC
Chambersburg PA
CBHW071013260726

48661CB00007B/2943